ISBN: 979-8-218-84506-3

Cover design by Zoë Klimek
Illustrations by Zoë Klimek and Karen Kilbourne-Thiel

Printed in the United States of America

First Edition

Disclaimer:
This book is intended for informational and educational purposes only. It is not a substitute for professional medical advice, diagnosis, or treatment. Always consult with a qualified healthcare provider regarding any questions or conditions related to your health or well-being.

Foreword

Written with love by Jayda Lee Jean

Women, we are connected by blood, through the all-encompassing womb. Everything I do, every sip of freedom I drink, is for you, sisters. We are connected by blood; We are one.

Zoë and I's friendship has been shaped and rooted deep through its own cycles and rhythms. A friendship that moves like a tide with the moon... inevitable. We were destined to awaken each other's Truth and the Truth, holding witness to becoming. Through many moons, we were beside each other, watching a sister shape shift, soften, harden, shed, and cultivate lived wisdom and, most importantly, come into Wombanhood. Together, we questioned the systems that infiltrate and blind many of us. We broke free together- Zoë, one wing & I, the other. Raw and truthful, our friendship has been a faithful mirror and a road back home again and again.

I have watched Zoë move through seasons of grief, blossoming, and fierce reclamation. The Earth breathes her. In the vibrant cradling greenscapes of Hawaii, I watched a divine spark in her flicker and take flame. An opening so tender and certain that even the plants seemed to lean in. On that sacred land, clarity settled into her bones. There are no accidents; even our initials were engraved on the land, the path opened here. The plants chose her, this work chose her, and she chose it back with a YES so steady it sounded like an ancient drum of knowing.

Zoë is a true Taurus, Earth tough and rooted, with tenderness that does not apologize. A flower in human form, offering forward wisdom that has lain dormant for too long, that reawakened through her awakening. She allowed her curiosity to guide her. She stripped herself bare and became so open to what was truly meant for her. She had, and continues to have and hold the courage to walk a path that is solely her own. There is something to be said about the women who are able to get naked enough and meet Truth. In this constant act of surrender, lives devotion.

Cyclical living is not merely a theory; It is an art you learn by doing, through devotion. It is a steady re-membering. The phases of the moon, the rise and fall of seasons, and the pulse of your own body are not separate things; They are a luminous conversation. Zoë guides and holds space without filling it for you; She trusts that you, too, are capable of remembering how to tend to your rhythm.

This book matters because we are one, and one by one, as we return to our bodies' wisdom, we set another sister free. We walk another sister home to drink from the cosmic, all-connected womb. The power of return is messy, but messy medicine shakes you awake unapologetically.

I lived numb and dependent on birth control for so many years, from age fifteen to twenty-one. In Hawaii, rooted on the Big Island, the land offered me the gift of courage to let it go and come home. In the past three years, I have come to know the power of my bleed, and I have cultivated so much respect for my body and the ways it communicates with me intelligently as a womb holder. There is nothing weak about your bleed or the sensitivity and changes that come with it. There is great power in it. The energetic work that is happening as you bleed is profound; You shed for your community, circles, loved ones, the collective, and your ancestors. As women, we are inherently energy workers. All that no longer serves is released through our blood. There is wisdom dripping down your legs and knowledge that is needed by the world that comes from you. You can't hold it, hear it, or translate it if you plug it up or turn it off. The earth needs you, and your connection to your womb, your sisters, too, and your brothers. Let us celebrate the fertile edges of our own becoming. The most revolutionary thing you can do is return to the wisdom of your blood.

Reading this book is an act of rewilding. Zoë's wisdom is a permission slip out of disconnection, into sovereign connection. You're likely here because you're curious, angry, weary, or hopeful. You've landed in gentle hands. This is wisdom that has been lived by Zoë herself and all of her sisters who walk this path with her. Practices tested in both sweetness and sorrow, and rituals that are simple enough but also so deep that they change the way you move through the world. You're crossing a threshold into the sacred... sacred shedding, planting, rising, resting, and knowing.

All necessary, and all Holy.

Treat these pages as an altar: with reverence, with an honest inventory of your needs, and with the soft courage to try something new. Let them teach you to translate the language of your own flesh. Know these pages are humming and pulsing with possibilities.

May Zoë's words meet you like a sister's long hug, steadying you into the moment, deepening your breath, and slowing you into a luminous return.

I love you until the Earth stops turning, my sweet and dearest sister, Zoë. I am honored to walk beside you, to learn from you, and to love you. Thank you, with all that I am.

With love,
Jayda Lee Jean

Table of Contents

Her-Story, not His-Story

Menses is Latin for month. *Mene* was the Ancient Greek word for "Moon" and even "Menstruation." When we look back at the language used to describe our cyclical nature, it is the root of time, and the Moon is a reflection of our internal clocks.

The first moon calendars date back to 28,000 B. C. Around 48 B.C., Julius Caesar decided to switch to the 12-month calendar (The Julian Calendar) after he visited Egypt and fell in love with Egyptian science. This new calendar system started in March. That month was named after the War God, Mars. He then named his birth month July after himself and August after his successor Augustus. Pope Gregory XIII realized the 12 months didn't align with the Solar Year, and so Leap Years were added in 1582 to make up for the miscalculation. This was the birth of the "Gregorian Calendar," which we still follow today.

The Solar Year is 365 days long. The Lunar Year is 354 days long and follows the 13 moon phases within the astrological wheel. This book serves as a guide to a basic understanding of our Cycle, and the journal section on Page 41 is intended to be followed for the Lunar Year. By tracking your Cycle under these moons, you may notice common themes with the cosmic energy and the moon phases above.

Your menstrual cycle is nothing to be ashamed of, as a lack of understanding within modern culture may make us feel. The red thread connects us to our bloodlines and all the women of the Earth- past, present, and future. It is your birthright to have access to its power. By following your own internal rhythm, you have the ability to tap into so much more of your powerful, Divine, Femininity. Following your natural rhythm allows you access to your True nature. Living in tune with your ebb and flow allows you to honor your body's call to rest and action. Connecting with your inner seasons is a powerful practice that allows us women to feel more deeply connected to the Earth and her sacred cycles. We can find more peace, surrender, and trust when we stop resisting what our body is telling us. With our Wombs as the compass for our lives, we see the ability to generate new beginnings cycle after cycle. Our menstrual blood is the only blood not shed through violence and holds sacred codes to our destiny.

Back in the days without electricity, the women of the village synced up with the New Moon or Full Moon. This dark-moon void, or bright reflection, was a time that was acknowledged as sacred. The women of the village would all gather together with their prayers and honor this period of darkness or illumination. Together, they would hold the weight of the Village. In Modern times, we are constantly exposed to things that are intentionally keeping us separate from our hormones, cycles, community, and sisterhood. Instead of bleeding together across the world under the New Moon and Full Moons, we are scattered across the moons, and some women even without a cycle. We now bear the weight of our villages on our own. This speaks to our Strength and power, but is not how we were meant to live.

With that said, I invite you to pause, connect to your breath, feel this next prayer in your heart and womb, and envision a world where we are all back in sync:

I pray that we can return to our cycles and restore the inherent balance within and all around us. I pray we can return to our organic template without disruption to our sacred hormones. I pray for a world that honors the Earth and Women's Cycles, Feminine nature, and respects our Power. And so it is.

Being a woman with a cycle is an incredible blessing. The average woman has roughly 450-500 periods in her lifetime, assuming no pregnancy, breastfeeding, or other cycle interruptions. That is 450-500 opportunities to embrace life and death in the beautiful body you were gifted; So many opportunities to shed the layers of all that we carry as women. Each body is unique, and so all information in here is for educational purposes and is to be used as a compass to point you in the direction of your own innate wisdom and truth. The rest is up to you to decipher what your body is sharing with you about its preferences and experiences.

The average cycle can be anywhere from 21-36 days. 70-80% of women cycle through 26-30 day periods. This varies with nutrition, stress, lifestyle, and energetic cycles. Your cycle has its own intelligence and is cycling WITH you in this life. It is safe to trust its rhythm through the seasons. It is on your side, supporting your energetic, physical, and emotional ebbs and flows.

If you asked any doctor, Menstrual, Follicular, Ovulation, and Luteal are the common medical terms that would be used to describe our phases. I feel that using the language of Internal Seasons rather than the medical terms helps grasp a deeper understanding of how the body is shifting. We can then begin to create safety in trusting our seasons as we are already practicing it externally on Earth. It reminds us that we are not separate from this planet. We aren't just ON it, we ARE it.

Saying, "I'm experiencing my Inner Winter," is more descriptive of what we are truly experiencing physically, energetically, and emotionally, rather than calling it our "Period." This term, truthfully, is a period of deep medicine, but was named after a time when our Moontimes/Inner Winter/Bleed (all used interchangeably) was looked at as a bloody period of illness and dis-ease. I have used the medicalized terms throughout this guide as some may already be familiar with this language. I intend to provide alternative verbiage to rewrite the script of how we interact and honor our Sacred Cycles.

In a world that's default operating system is "A Man's World," living in a 24 hour cycle following the sun vs a 28 day female cycle following the moon, everything feels so fast-paced. We were not built to operate this way. No wonder we're collectively overwhelmed, anxious, and disconnected. There's not enough time to slow down. It is up to us to live the Truth of our bodies and choose to slow down to embrace sacred rest.

Within each 21-36 day cycle, you are going through all four seasons. With each season comes its own unique call to action, nutritional needs, emotions, and physical changes. It is nice to know these ranges, as you can begin to attune to what you're feeling and where you're at in your cycle. Your Inner Winter Phase (Menstruation) may range from 1 to 7 days. Inner Spring (Follicular) ranges 7-12 days. Inner Summer (Ovulation) ranges 3 to 5 days. Inner Autumn (Luteal) ranges 10-17 days. These numbers can vary with your rhythm and can be discovered by tracking your cycle as laid out in Page 41 and 44. As you begin to ride your cycle, you will find what's normal for you. I invite you to track your cycle for at least 13 moons (New Moon to Full Moon).

Organizing your life around your cycle can unlock a new level of self-acceptance, energy management, rest, and productivity in the Feminine way. Living from this place of flow can also support your heart-centered dreams, visions, goals, and business. While results may vary, many women start to feel the benefits of cycle syncing after one to three cycles. Consistent practice is key, as understanding the different phases of your cycle takes time. Brick by brick, you'll begin to lay a new template. This will be an ever-evolving practice.

This process requires dedication and discipline. This form of discipline is an act of self-love. Initially, you may find it frustrating or challenging. Give yourself grace, kindness, and compassion. The young girl within is learning with you too. It is normal to feel bitterness towards the systems for not teaching us this. Acknowledge and validate these feelings. It is your choice and responsibility to alchemize and reclaim this power for yourself. Think of all those who will now learn from you because you chose this path of dedication.

Returning to the Matriarchal way of living brings balance and harmony back into our lives. It involves living with this internal flow, which ultimately impacts our external worlds. We were put on this Earth to live with her. We are just as much Earth as she is us. It is time to stop resisting the seasons we are experiencing.

This reconnection allows us to be more accepting of the Self in an external world where the male's Circadian Rhythm is the dominant flow of life. This does not match up with how we cycling women feel internally, leaving us feeling burnt out, not enough, and scrambling to keep up. By attuning to our inner rhythms, we can understand the Earth's seasons more deeply, which guides us back to a deeper knowing of trust sourced from within that WE are the Divine timing. There is a reason for every season on this beautiful planet. There is a time for life, death, and rebirth; A time to grow and expand; A time to flourish and shine; A time to shed layers; A time to go inward and reflect. The same rhythm happens within YOU during each INternal Moon Cycle you experience.

Embracing cyclical living is the biggest act of sacred rebellion and service to those before and after us. Things were not always this way, and once again, we will return to our inherent magic. I've been blessed to be able to embrace this, and you can too. You are the creator of your own life. Set your boundaries and watch things fall into place. The Earth and Cosmos are conspiring with you. Remember, the power that these elements hold is far stronger than the man-made layer of social conditioning.

DISCLAIMER: This guide is not intended to initiate or prevent pregnancy, or give medical advice. It is simply a supportive tool that invites you to attune your own inner rhythm. Each body and cycle is different. I intend to share the framework of what has worked for me and my sisters alike.

Thank you for being here. Thank you for choosing to acknowledge the Power that lies within your Womb. Thank you for listening to the Call and choosing to do the work. Thank you for showing up for the ancestors before and after you. Thank you for showing up for the Sisters who are already in the Village practicing this and weaving the web of Remembrance across the globe. Each Woman who chooses to honor herself makes this web stronger. This work is so much bigger than you can even imagine and also directly benefits you. It is so rewarding to know yourself this deeply. It is an endless portal of Wisdom. The fruits of this labor will bring abundance to you and everyone on this Earth.

Fractured Femininity-The Cost of Birth Control

Margaret Sanger, a woman tied to the interest of Eugenics, existed during the time of WW1. She worked very hard to legalize birth control. The first case studies were done in Puerto Rico where 135 women used birth control for 12 months and were not told any of the risks associated with the contraceptive. Out of the 135 women, five died. One of the deaths was by suicide and was claimed to not be from birth control. When birth control sought FDA approval, many women came forward but were unable to tell the truth of the discomfort and side effects they had out of fear.

In the 1930's, slave hospitals in the United States became the next space for experimentation. Women, especially of color, were told they couldn't recieve government housing or food stamps unless they got the Long Acting Contraceptive, an implant that was unable to be removed. Women were also told they were having their tubes tied, but later found out they had their tubes cut, rendering them, and it was irreversible and were now sterilized.

In the beginning of the birth control movement, no labeling with side effects was provided. Barbara Seaman, author of The Doctors' Case Against The Pill, is an important figure to note for her work during the time of the Women's Health Movement in the 1970's. Her writings prompted Senate hearings in 1970 that led to a warning label on birth control and influenced companies to lower the estrogen doses due to their harmful side effects. The labeling evolved to a slight increase in warning with the major focus being on blood clots. Birth control now comes with pages of small printed warnings.

Yaz was the first birth control FDA approved and released to the public. Loryna was a generic version of Yaz that contained the same ingredients and hormones. Both have had multiple lawsuits against their products being stated as the cause of death for many young, healthy women.

"We're looking to medical technology for liberation and that means whatever contraception comes on the market we defend it. It's so tied into our freedom but at what cost?" *The Business of Birth Control.*

The revolution of a simple pill has now become a multi-billion dollar company. "We're not setting women free, we're setting them up for disease." Erika Schwartz MD. The FDA only approves drugs for two weeks and then it is up to the manufacturers. These drug companies are majorly profiting and killing our women for their gain and convenience.

35% of women on it are prescribed for PMS reasons. 1:10 women suffer from endometriosis. 1:10 women suffer from poly-cystic ovary syndrome (PCOS). Birth control is the number one culprit of fibroids, PCOS, blood clots, pulmonary embolisms, endometriosis, and infertility. A heavy cycle is a symptom of the root cause of fibroids; It is the result of excess estrogen which is triggered by stress, diet, and pollutants. Chemical pollutants, such as birth control, is the number one factor of excess estrogen. Many believe the pill is the greatest invention but it's harmful and in some cases is lethal.

Hormonal birth control turns off organic hormonal flow and utilizes synthetic hormones. In the standard pill-form of birth control there are three weeks of the synthetic hormones; The fourth week is a sugar pill that imitates the drop in hormones we'd experience naturally before our bleed. This is a withdrawal bleed, not a true experience of menstruation. Hormonal birth control turns off ovulation. Regular ovulation, organically without the use of birth control, is how we make our estrogen and progesterone. These hormones are critical to our health and well-being. Hormones have many benefits for our bodies such as: bone, breast, and brain development, metabolism, mood regulation, libido, and they support cardiovascular health now and into the future.

12 million women in America have used birth control. A high number of women have reported the following symptoms while using birth control: painful sex, low libido, migraine headaches, nutrient deficiency, insomnia, clitoral shrinkage, partner attraction*, pheromone alteration, stroke, heart attack, heart disease, anxiety, depression, panic attacks, infertility, weight gain, and diabetes. Hormonal birth control causes a dampened stress response in the brain, which increases cortisol. This dampened condition causes memory issues, brain fog, and decreases the ability to learn, retain information, and deal with stress. A study done in Denmark by Dr. Ojvind Lindegaard, found an 80% increased risk of depression for women who started hormonal birth control between the ages 15-19. There have been no long-term studies done on mental and reproductive health. This is a concern, especially for the girls who are starting birth control younger than ever before.

*Partner attraction: There are many stories about women going off birth control and then finding they are unhappy with who they chose as a mate. The MHC complex (Major Histocompatibility Complex) is a group of genes that gives us data about the other's immune system and genetic capability, but this is compromised when on birth control. This leads to disruption of our natural selection.

Women shouldn't have to change who they are in order to protect themselves from pregnancy," Sarah E. Hill, PhD, author of *Your Brain on Birth Control*.

With all of that being said, what are we allowing to be done to us and our inherent nature? It is critical we return to our organic templates for the sake of our bodies, spirits, children, families. Freedom is informed consent and the choice to do what we wish with that information. True liberation is being able to live freely in our bodies, embrace the seasons we internally experience, and use our Power as God intended.

"Birth control was legalized in the 1960's for women to take fertility into their own hands. Oral contraceptives allowed us to control when we were ovulating and not disclose when we were sexually active. It opened doors for us to be able to work and pursue our dreams. Birth control was looked at as revolutionary, and as "The Great Liberator," paraphrased from the 2021 documentary, *The Business of Birth Control*. Birth Control served its purpose back in those days. We regained control of our bodies but it was still a form of suppression at the expense of fracturing our organic nature.

In my experience, birth control did the opposite of liberate me. It was a choice made rooted in shame, fear and avoidance. It suppressed my intuition and I gave up my sovereignty to embrace my biggest super power: being a Cycling Woman. I missed out on 78 periods over the six years I was on birth control. That's 78 opportunities to have been able to alchemize all the valuable lessons of maturity I endured in my late teens.

I do not share this to shame others who chose or continue to choose birth control. Instead, to offer a perspective on the myriad obstacles that stand in the way of full body autonomy and authenticity. We have been deprived of the pure magic that we are. When we don't have all the facts, we are unable to make informed decisions.

I share my story here because I feel so deeply that this invention came about for us to be further separated from our true nature, and the time is now to return to our organic template. Since writing this book, my mother and I have connected deeply over this topic. By bringing this forth, I've gotten to share this information with her that neither she nor my grandma never received. This work is healing many generations before and after me and is not intended to place blame on any of these women. In reclaiming this wisdom for myself, it's being reclaimed for us all.

When I was 15, I remember telling my mom I wanted to start taking birth control because I had "bad PMS cramps," but truthfully I was becoming sexually active and was uneducated on when I could actually become pregnant. I was never taught that we have multiple phases. This was more than just bleeding and not bleeding. I made this choice out of fear and lack of body awareness. I set a reminder on my phone each evening to take my birth control for four years straight. Week four of my pill pack was the "sugar pill." My doctor told me I could occasionally skip this week and start the next pack if I wanted to skip my period. I did this more than occasionally; I did it almost every month. I wore it as a badge of honor that I didn't have to "deal" with my period each month. I do not advise this now!

Towards the end of the four years, I was intuitively questioning if this was messing with my fertility. When I asked my doctor about this, she told me no. I had trouble with the consistency so I decided to switch to an IUD and continued with birth control. In reflection, this choice was made out of avoidance of a responsibility, which was to take true control of my fertility. I put it in the hands of my doctor, literally. That choice resulted in spotting every day for over eight months. I had it in for just shy of two years when I decided it wasn't worth the discomfort any longer.

Birth Control free, my doctors shared the Fertility Awareness Method (FAM) and introduced me to an app to track my cycle. I did this pretty passively until one day, I really started paying attention to the suggestions offered for diet and lifestyle. I dove down this rabbit hole and never turned back. My whole life has completely shifted and this book is my life's practice. I share this from one sister to another.

Our power is Ours to reclaim through Cyclical living, and is the key to restoring the balance and relationship with Earth. Birth Control is just that- controlling birth by adjusting our body's natural processes which is incredibly harmful to the miracle of an organic Woman. We are not meant to be tamed!

Meditation for Cyclical Connection and Remembrance

I suggest reading this aloud while recording in your own voice memos so you can replay it and drop in anytime you'd like to do this meditation:

Find a quiet place to sit where you won't be interrupted. Take a moment to close your eyes. Notice your breath without trying to control it. Is it deep or light? Notice your heartbeat. Notice where your mind wants to wander. Gently bring it back to the present. Feel the blood pulsing through your body and down to your womb. Your womb has its own rhythm and beat. Imagine a root emerging from the base of your spine, grounding deep into the Earth. Feel how this is connecting you to the Earth's heartbeat and her sacred cycles. Now, imagine yourself in a circle of women, a group of dear sisters who are also rooted and cycling through the seasons. See your grandmothers, your mother, sisters, daughters, and granddaughters. Feel the sense of community in knowing they are all moving through the waves with you. Envision the circle growing bigger, all the women and ancestors of the Earth sitting in this circle with the dark, New Moon and stars above you. Feel the warmth of the fiery sun inside you, the air coming in and out of you, the waters moving internally, and the Earth beneath you. Together, you begin to weave a web between you. This web gets stronger and stronger with every strand. Feel the hum of your hearts. Your cycles begin to sync up, and you feel held by one another. You can feel all the seasons swirling, happening inside and outside of you. In the stillness of your being amidst these forces, a loud collective prayer goes out. A prayer we can live in a world where we honor ourselves by putting our cyclical needs first. A prayer for deeper compassion and understanding that each season we move through can be fully accepted and embraced by us and the outside world. A prayer for strength and courage to share this wisdom with our daughters, granddaughters, and all the children and men. Lastly, a prayer for humanity that we can come back to the inner knowing we all have deep inside that we are not meant to live in a world where we push against this nature, and that balance can be restored when we respect and honor this way of being. Settle into this feeling and know that by choosing this path to follow your cyclical nature, we are healing ourselves and Earth. Placing your hands on your heart and womb, come back to your conscious breath and take a moment to notice any shifts that have taken place within your body. Notice the feelings of strength and courage that you now have woven into your field. When you are ready, slowly return the sensations in your fingers and toes with some gentle movement. Gently open your eyes and re-emerge yourself back into the physical reality. Know that you are so loved and supported in this cyclical journey that you have begun.

Journal Prompts to Explore Your Relationship With Your Cycle

- Recall and journal your story of Menarche (your first bleed). What happened before, during, after?

- Were your feelings validated and met with patience and understanding?

- What messages (spoken or unspoken) did you receive about menstruation growing up? How did they shape the way you relate to your body?

- What parts of your wild nature were tamed, shamed, or silenced as you grew into womanhood? Were you told you were "too much"?

- In what ways have you feared or resisted the wild within yourself? What would it mean to welcome her home— bleeding, fierce, and free?

- Create a new message for your inner maiden (use empowering, beautiful wording to rewire and reclaim your womanhood) Repeat this message over & over

- How do you feel when women talk about their monthly bleed? And do you talk openly about your cycle with others? Why or why not?

- How does your Moontime (Inner Winter/Menstrual Phase) make you feel? What is this relationship like?

Menarche-Honoring the Initiation

Menarche, is a term used to describe a girl's first menstrual bleed, marking the beginning of her reproductive years. It is an important time of initiation from Girlhood to Womanhood. In cultures across the world, such as Native American and Hindu, Menarche is a time of celebration. Rituals are held to honor this major transitional time and vary across cultures.

In Muslim cultures and countries such as Africa and the United States, Menarche is not something that is commonly honored. Unfortunately, menstruation has a harmful stereotype around it, such as an "impurity" and a curse. This stigma leads to shame, discrimination, and even violence. In some cultures, women are not allowed to attend social events, touch objects such as food or water, use sanitary products, or be taught about proper menstrual hygiene.

Like most girls in America, we receive the "talk" in health class. I vividly remember the school nurse holding up a glass measuring cup with some red Gatorade in it, saying, "This is how much blood you shed during your period." The sixth grade girls came up with the "code word," *Peaches,* to use to talk about our Moontime. It was as if saying "blood" was something to hide and be ashamed of. The lack of education also led to fear of when that day would come. "Am I going to just bleed out in the middle of class!?" Fear was instilled in us before we even had the opportunity to decide what it meant to us.

When we don't acknowledge menstruation for what it is, there is a disconnect from our true organic nature. When we choose to recognize this transition, harmony is restored within ourselves and the Earth. Being a Womban is a blessing and holds sacred responsibility in following our rhythm. It is what makes us different and is something to be proud of. Mother Earth doesn't hide her nature; She embraces it. We are not meant to be contained!

Depending on the young woman and how she's feeling about this transition, it could be nice to have a "First Moon Party." This can look many different ways, such as a nice meal, a sleepover with her girlfriends, an all-out party with red velvet cake and decorations, or a simple, small ritual of acknowledgment like lighting a red candle and creating an altar. It's never too late to host a celebration! After learning this, I created a ritual as part of my 25th birthday party. No matter your age, this is still a piece of you that deserves to be honored.

Now, I invite you to be open to the guidance of this book to help reframe the language of what it means to be a Cyclical Womban. Allow the illusions of shame to dissolve and be recreated. This book is how we should've been taught to live with our cycles. This book is for US, and together we are reclaiming our POWER.

Reading Your Basal Body Temperature

Your basal body temperature (BBT) is your body's lowest resting temperature and is measured after resting for at least four hours. Ideally, it's taken just as you wake up and before you get out of bed. This form of tracking helps you understand when you're ovulating and fertile. A Basal Thermometer is different from the average thermometer as it shows two decimal places vs. one. It can be found online or at a local drugstore. Take your temperature and record it in your log daily as provided in Pages 42 and 44.

This temperature should rise .5-0.1°F when you're ovulating. During pregnancy, progesterone levels remain high and cause a sustained increase in BBT. Progesterone is one of the primary hormones that sustains pregnancy. If implantation doesn't occur, this temperature should fall back down to your regular temperature. Since the increase in BBT occurs at or after ovulation, the fertile period begins several days before you notice a drop in temperature. In simpler terms, your temperature will stay high and consistent if you do become pregnant or fall back down after ovulation if you are not. You can become pregnant in the week leading up to the peak in temperature.

Keep in mind that while the BBT method can help track your cycle and fertile window, your body temperature can be affected by many external factors and relies on tracking very small changes over time. Charting your temperature over time can provide information about the timing of your cycle to predict fertility in future months. A chart is provided for you to track your BBT on Page 44.

This temperature can also tell you about your thyroid health. If your baseline daily temperature is lower than 97.8°F consistently, that may signal hypothyroid (an under-active thyroid). Thyroid health is important because this endocrine gland creates the hormones that regulate body temperature, heart rate, metabolism, energy levels, and play an important role in the menstrual cycle. Imbalances can lead to various health concerns, so low temperatures should be discussed with a medical professional.

Reading Your Vaginal Release

The Cervical Mucus Method, The Ovulation Method, or The Billings Method

It is best not to rely on the Cervical Mucus Method solely for birth control unless you have already tracked this for at least one cycle. It is also more effective to use this method in conjunction with taking your Basal Body temperature daily. Using these two together is called the Symptothermal Method. Throughout this book, you will notice I refer to Cervical Mucus as vaginal release, release, fluid release. This is to help reframe the language of the sacred fluids that are speaking to us from our bodies.

To track this way, you will need to check your release daily and write it down in a log. Use the journal section and/or chart on Pages 42 and 44. There are a few ways you can check this release: Before you urinate for the first time of the day, wipe your vulva with clean tissue and evaluate the color and texture; check your underwear for color and texture; Alternatively, insert clean fingers, swipe, feel the texture and notice the color. The best way to feel the consistency of your discharge is to rub it between your thumb and index finger. Note everything you notice about your release in a journal daily: your period days, dry days, wet days, sticky days, cloudy days, and slippery days.

Inner Winter (Menstrual): Blood flow will cover the fluid release, so it is considered the "unsafe days" to have ejaculatory sex if you are intending to avoid pregnancy. Right after the blood flow ends, there should be about three to four days where there is no fluids released. These few days are considered "safe days" since the dry release is not the fertile soil needed for reproduction to occur. Refer to Page 23 to learn how to read your menstrual blood.

Inner Spring (Follicular): As your egg starts to ripen, the body creates more fluids. This release normally appears cloudy, yellow, or white and feels sticky. You may also notice this release around the opening of your Vagina. These days are less safe for ejaculatory sex as the soil becomes more fertile during this phase, and sperm can live internally for about five days waiting around for the egg to drop. If your cycle is shorter, this process happens more quickly than in the longer cycle, and ejaculatory sex is not recommended if intended to prevent pregnancy.

Inner Summer (Ovulation): Just before Ovulation, you should have the most fluid. It should appear clear and feel slippery like an egg white when stretched between your fingers. These slippery days are when you are most fertile, so they are "unsafe" days for ejaculatory sex. If you're trying to conceive, then this is the time to act! This release should last about four days, leading up to and at the time of ovulation.

Inner Fall (Luteal) After the peak of ovulation, you may notice far less fluid. It will become sticky and cloudy again and eventually go away, leading to more dry days preceding your Moontime (Bleed).

Other Colors:
- **Clumpy and white** release could be a sign of a yeast infection, along with other symptoms like itching and irritation

- **Yellow or green** release could be a sign of an infection, especially if a foul smell accompanies it

- **Gray** release could be a sign of bacterial vaginosis (BV). Another common sign of BV is a strong fishy smell

- **Pink or brown** release could be a sign that your Bleed is beginning or ending, and a bit of blood has mixed with your fluid. However, if you also feel pain, itching, or irritation, this could be a sign of an infection.

If any of these occur, consult with a trusted medical professional or trained herbalist.

Reading Your Menstrual Blood

The practice of reading your blood can tell you many things about what's going on in your body.

It is normal for your blood to range from pink to bright red, then dark red to dark brown. These color changes occur with the day of menstruation and the strength of your flow. The faster your flow, the brighter red it will appear. As your blood is exposed to oxygen, it becomes a darker brown color the longer it is outside your blood cells. This process is called oxidation.

The light pink is a dilution of the blood as it's being mixed with your fluid release and is common at the beginning of your Moontime. A bright strawberry red blood flow appears a day after your bleed and indicates a strong flow occurring. The color shifting to a darker red indicates the blood flow slowing down as it's exposed to more oxygen before the blood is released from the body. A brown tint comes at the end of your Moontime as it takes even more time leaving the uterus with more oxidation occurring.

- A thicker, clottier, heavier flow may suggest stress and/or off-diet
- A cloudy bleed may suggest malnourishment during the last cycle
- A bright red flow that is darker and then lighter suggests a healthy, balanced flow in the previous cycle

Tracking cycle length and any symptoms can help you spot patterns and get used to what's normal for your body. Understanding and applying the teachings of blood color can show you where you need to make adjustments in your life.

The Cherokee believe menstrual blood is a source of Feminine strength and has the power to destroy enemies. In some cultures, it is seen as a symbol of creativity, fertility, and life-giving power. An ancient Hopi prophecy says, "When the women give their blood back to the earth, men will come home from war and Earth shall find peace."

One practice that I really look forward to each month to connect with this energy is collecting my blood during the second day of my bleed (or when your flow is strongest). I collect this blood by using a menstrual cup and then pour it into a mason jar. I will then use it for a face mask, dilute and water my plants, or use it as paint for my art. Using my blood in these ways has supported me in deepening my connection to my womb and her power. I also love the energetics behind it because when we bleed, we are shedding all the patterns and emotional toxins from the previous cycle. Wearing my blood on my face feels like a power move in knowing I sifted through all the gunk and have physically shed it all.

Working With Your Menstrual Blood

Menstrual blood has been found to hold an immense amount of stem cells and is not "dirty," like we are led to believe. I have supported healing my skin conditions by utilizing my menstrual blood topically each month on troubled areas. Applying the blood as a face mask always leaves my skin radiant and I feel like such a warrior wearing it which is why I call it "The Warrior Face Mask." (This is an activity noted in Internal Winter phase on Page 30 and the Cycle Overview Chart on Pages 43.)

My plants began to thrive when I shared this with them, and I believe it's a beautiful way to alchemize what's been shed, allowing me to watch it transform through working with the plant's elements. Using it in my art is also a beautiful way to work with and alchemize the energetics of what I've gone through in the previous cycle.

Commercial tampons and pads are loaded with toxins and endocrine disruptors, which are very harmful to our bodies. Pads are actually worse than tampons. I choose to wear period underwear and "Free-Bleed" because I have found that my cramps lessen, and I feel a clearer release of the blood being shed. A brand I love and have invested in is Wild Moon. Their material is soft, breathable, and they don't treat their products with PFAs, which are endocrine disruptors. They offer various styles for different flows and also have a youth line. Rinsing them out when I'm done also feels so sacred and intentional in physically washing away that which I am no longer carrying. The intentional time spent rinsing also slows me down to see I am, in fact, bleeding and shouldn't be running around like a chicken with my head cut off, trying to keep up with the Patriarchal way of living.

Blood Magick Rituals involve using your menstrual blood in a sacred way. By connecting to your intuition, find the intention for your ritual: To break down a taboo? Heal something? Create a boundary? Manifest something? Release an old habit or break a pattern? Celebrate the moon or your cycle? Once you have your intention, create an altar with things that are symbolic for you, such as candles, crystals, or ornaments. Call in any ancestors, spirit allies, or elements through a prayer or meditation to support you in this ritual. Offer gratitude to your body and blood for this gift. Place your blood on the altar, draw a symbol or sigil, incorporate it in spellwork, or any other way you feel called to that aligns with your intention. When you feel complete, close the ritual, ground yourself, thank all those whom you've called in, and release any energy that was invoked. There is no wrong way to do this, and it is purely up to you and your intuition!

Skin Cycling

Winter

~Low Progesterone: Low Oil Production
~Low Estrogen: Low Skin Barrier function
~Skin is sensitive and easily inflamed
~Facial Steam with dried or fresh herbs such as Chamomile, Lavender, Calendula, White Willow Bark to calm inflammation and redness
~Focus on gentle exfoliation, hydrosols, hydrating moisturizers, oils, ceramides, hyaluronic acid, and The Warrior Face Mask

Summer

~Estrogen peaks: skin is glowing
~Use gentle exfoliators
~Great season to book a facial
~Deep cleanse pores to prep for sebum uptick on cycle days 16-17
~Make a face mask with clay and mix in powdered herbs such as Rose (cools the skin) and Cedar (cleanses and exfoliates)
~Clays:

- Oily/Acne Prone Skin: Moroccan Red Clay or White Kaolin Clay which unclogs pores and absorbs excess oil
- Normal to Oily Skin: Try Bentonite Clay to draw out impurities and tighten skin
- Sensitive/Reactive Skin: French Green Clay which detoxes and heals skin
- Pigmentation: Fuller's Earth Clay which draws out excess sebum and lightens skin
- Aging Skin: Rhassoul Clay which hydrates and revitalizes skin

~Make Rose tea and freeze in ice cubes to rub on the face in the morning for a cooling and toning effect

Spring

~Estrogen is increasing: skin is rebalancing
~Collagen, elastin, and hyaluronic acid levels rise
~Support cellular turnover: use retinols, Vitamin C, peptides, niacinamide, and sunscreen
~Maintain skin hydration and stimulate blood flow with facial roller or massages
~Face mask with warm Honey and Matcha to help hydrate and brighten the skin
~Facial Steam with dried or fresh herbs such as Lemon, Orange, and Alfalfa for their vitamin and mineral content
-

Autumn

~Higher levels of progesterone and testosterone increase sebum and oil production, causing hormonal breakouts
~Pores tighten up and skin swells, which causes the face to look more round or puffy.
~Focus on oil control: use salicylic acid and deep clean pores
~Exfoliate
~Facial Steam with dried or fresh herbs such as Eucalyptus, Peppermint, Rosemary, Goldenrod for excess oil

Yoni Steaming

The term *"Yoni"* comes from the Sanskrit word for female genitalia, the womb, and the vagina. It means *"sacred place"* and symbolizes our divine nature and its sacred portal to life. Yoni steaming is an ancient practice that brings a deeper sense of connection to self and your womb space. It may also be referred to as pelvic steaming or vaginal steaming among other terms.

Yoni steams are part of the Mayan healing lineage and are used mainly to cleanse the uterus when there are menstrual difficulties, after birth, and with menopause to completely clean the womb when finished bleeding. They are popular in Central America, India, Eastern Europe, and in Korea, where women commonly incorporate them as part of their self-care routines.

Yoni steaming offers us the opportunity to restore the disconnect from our female body, yoni/uterus, whether that be from birth, unsatisfying intimate experiences, trauma, abuse, surgeries, or cultural disconnect. Yoni steaming is a self-love practice that restores health and balance to your physical feminine cycles, eases the transition through life phases, unlocks the intimate magic of your womb, and releases toxic emotions such as stress, tension, and stagnation.

Steams can be used to support energetic clearing of the womb, shedding of the lingering residue from the last bleed, a preventative and support for menstrual or ovulation cramps, preparation for the incoming bleed by opening up the womb space, rebalancing pH after intercourse, conditions of the womb such as UTI's, healing after childbirth, or to support the womb in fertility. DO NOT steam if you are ovulating, pregnant, bleeding (menstruating), or have an IUD.

Essentially, herbs are brewed in a steam pot, and the container is placed under you or under your open-seated chair. Blankets and sheets are wrapped around your torso to create a kind of sweat lodge for your lower torso. Sit and receive the moist warmth of the healing steam. It enters your body directly through your yoni and penetrates to your uterus, pelvis, and even up through a deep central channel connecting to your heart, so you can reconnect with your feminine body. Setting an intention for clearing the womb space and calling in your ancestors can be a powerful ritual. I find it nice to light some candles, burn incense, and have a relaxing playlist on. Following the ritual, I feel recentered in my womb, and the steam makes me feel warm from the inside out.

Each herb has a different reaction to the tissue state. Tissue state can be described as Hot (Warming), Cold (Cooling), Damp (Moistening), or Dry (Drying). Depending on the tissue state, herbs can have a different effect on the body. UTIs and Inflammation are a Hot tissue state; Yeast is Hot and Damp; Irregular cycles, Ovulation, and Cysts are a Cold and Damp state. When choosing the herbs, you want to pick ones that have the opposite effect as the tissue state. It is important to tune into your womb to know how her tissue state is before gathering the correct herbs to Yoni Steam with. Below, I have listed some commonly used herbs and the way they affect the body. Many of them cross over in the categories, such as Rose can be Aromatic, Digestive, and Disinfecting.

Aromatic:
- Rose (Cooling, Moistening)
- Lemon (Cooling, Drying)
- Orange (Cooling, Moistening)
- Lavender (Warming, Moistening)
- Lemon Balm (Cooling, Drying)

Cleansing:
- Motherwort (Cooling, Drying)
- Red Clover (Cooling, Moistening)
- Calendula (Warming when steamed, Moistening)

Blood & Kidney Tonic:
- Nettle (Warming, Drying)
- Red Clover
- Rosemary- (Warming, Drying) is also antiseptic and helps with circulating out old fluids and blood. It purifies and stimulates the yoni and helps to reclaim and remember lost parts of yourself

Toning and Healing:
- Red Raspberry Leaf (Cooling, Drying)
- Motherwort
- Calendula-Helpful for tears and scar tissue
- Nettle

Disinfecting:
- Calendula
- Lavender- a sweet-smelling antiseptic and antibacterial herb with soothing and powerful cleansing properties for a healthy vaginal environment
- Lemon, Orange, Lemon Balm, Calendula

Digestive: There is a direct connection between the gut and the uterus.
- Dandelion-(Cooling, Drying) helps improve endocrine and reproductive health. It helps rid excess estrogen, sugars, and toxins of the body
- Mint (Cooling)
- Citrus Peels

Antispasmodic (Cramping):
- Lavender
- Red Raspberry Leaf
- Lemon Balm
- Calendula
- Red Clover

Bleeding With The Moon

Another layer of menstrual cycle awareness that can support a deeper understanding of what may be happening physically, emotionally, mentally, and spiritually is noticing what phase the Moon is in and where you are in your cycle.

The New Moon represents a time of introspection, rebirth, beginnings, transformation, and planting new seeds. The dark sky mirrors to us a blank slate. When your bleed starts on or around the New Moon, this is known as a White Moon Cycle. You would then be ovulating with the Full Moon–the Earth's most fertile time. This way of cycling is associated with the Mother archetype because this is the Earth's natural rhythm of life. The internal and external energies are in sync with the planet and then become magnified. Women who bleed during this time are said to be moving through a time where they are being asked to give more energy to themselves, turning inward and focusing on self-learning and inner growth instead of looking outward for a while.

The Full Moon represents a time of completion, release, purge, expansion, and reflection. Energy is heightened at this time and our intuition is illuminated. When your bleed starts at or around the Full Moon, this is known as the Red Moon Cycle. You would then be ovulating with the New Moon. Many moons ago, in ancient times, women who bled with the Full moon were seen as healers, witches, and priestesses because their energy was being asked to be focused on sacred circles within their community, teaching, and guiding others, rather than turning inward like the White Moon Cyclers. The Red Moon offers a deeper connection to our sexual energy and creativity.

The Waxing Moon represents a time of transition between the New and Full Moon. When your bleed starts during this time, it may indicate that you're going through a transitional phase in your life and it is referred to as the Pink Moon Cycle. The moon is shifting from darkness to lightness and translates in your body as a time where you are moving from a period of rest and coming into your power and strength.

The Waning Moon represents a time of transition between the Full and New Moon. When your bleed starts during this time, it is referred to as the Purple Moon Cycle. This indicates that you are moving through a transitional phase, but in the other direction. The moon is shifting from strength and power into a time of darkness and shadows. This translates in your body as a time where you're moving from outward expansion and being invited back into introspection.

In a woman's life, she may transition in and out of the White, Pink, Red, or Purple Moon Cycles. It is a dance with the Moon, inviting us to move through her rhythms and experience them for ourselves. Embrace your natural rhythms. There is wisdom in it all. You are a Cyclical Womban and you are sacred.

Internal Winter

The Menstrual Phase~ Reset and Restoration

Hormones: During this season, the Corpus Luteum drops the progesterone and triggers menstruation due to the egg not becoming fertilized. The lining of your uterus is being shed in this phase. Estrogen and testosterone are low here.

Cervical Release: Blood should flow from light pink to bright red to darker red to darker brown throughout your Moontime.

Do: Your Inner Winter is a call to slow all the way down and pause to reflect on what did and didn't work in the last cycle. Notice any resistance you have with slowing down. What is your relationship with rest? Notice how wound tight you may be and how long it takes you to drop into the stillness this season calls for. It is a great time for flow art, painting with your menstrual blood, and applying menstrual blood face masks. The Warrior face mask can feel very empowering and will have your skin absolutely glowing due to the high content of stem cells.

Move: It may feel nice to take a bath, journal, create art, practice breath work and meditation, take light walks, and incorporate gentle stretching to ease cramping in flows such as Yin Yoga or Menstrual Movement. Avoid inverted movement due to the gravitational pull and release of blood. In this phase, try to focus on activities that promote relaxation and release. Connect with the Moon, anoint yourself, practice divination, honor your ancestors, give your blood to the Earth, free-bleed, or create an altar to celebrate this phase.

Eat: The focus in this season is to replenish what is being lost through menstruation and to support the body during this process. Cook warm and easily digestible foods; Avoid cold foods, caffeine, and alcohol; Intake fiber-rich foods to support digestive health; Grounding root vegetables; B Vitamin-rich foods to support energy levels and mood; Omega-3 Fatty Acids to help with menstrual cramping and inflammation; Magnesium-rich foods to help with menstrual cramping and sleep; Iron-rich Foods to replenish iron lost during menstruation and prevent anemia.

Herbs: Red Clover, Nettle, Chamomile, Catnip, Cinnamon, Nutmeg, Turmeric, Ginger, Hawthorn, Cedar, Raspberry Leaf, Rose Petals, Orange Peel, Cloves, Skullcap, Passionflower, Fennel, Cacao, Milk Thistle, Oatstraw, Dandelion Root or Leaf, Linden, Damiana

Common Experiences: Cramping, bloating, emotional sensitivity, inflammation, fatigue, headaches, breast tenderness, and menstrual bleeding are all common experiences in this season. You may also feel extra introspective. I like to call this my "Moon Cocoon" time, where I tune the world out, turn inward to my internal landscape, and see what needs to be shed.

Archetype: The *Maiden* archetype is associated with this season. The *Maiden* embodies exploration, beginnings, curiosity, release, renewal, and preparation for what's to come. During menstruation, it is prime time for dreaming and visioning as your intuition and creative insights are heightened.

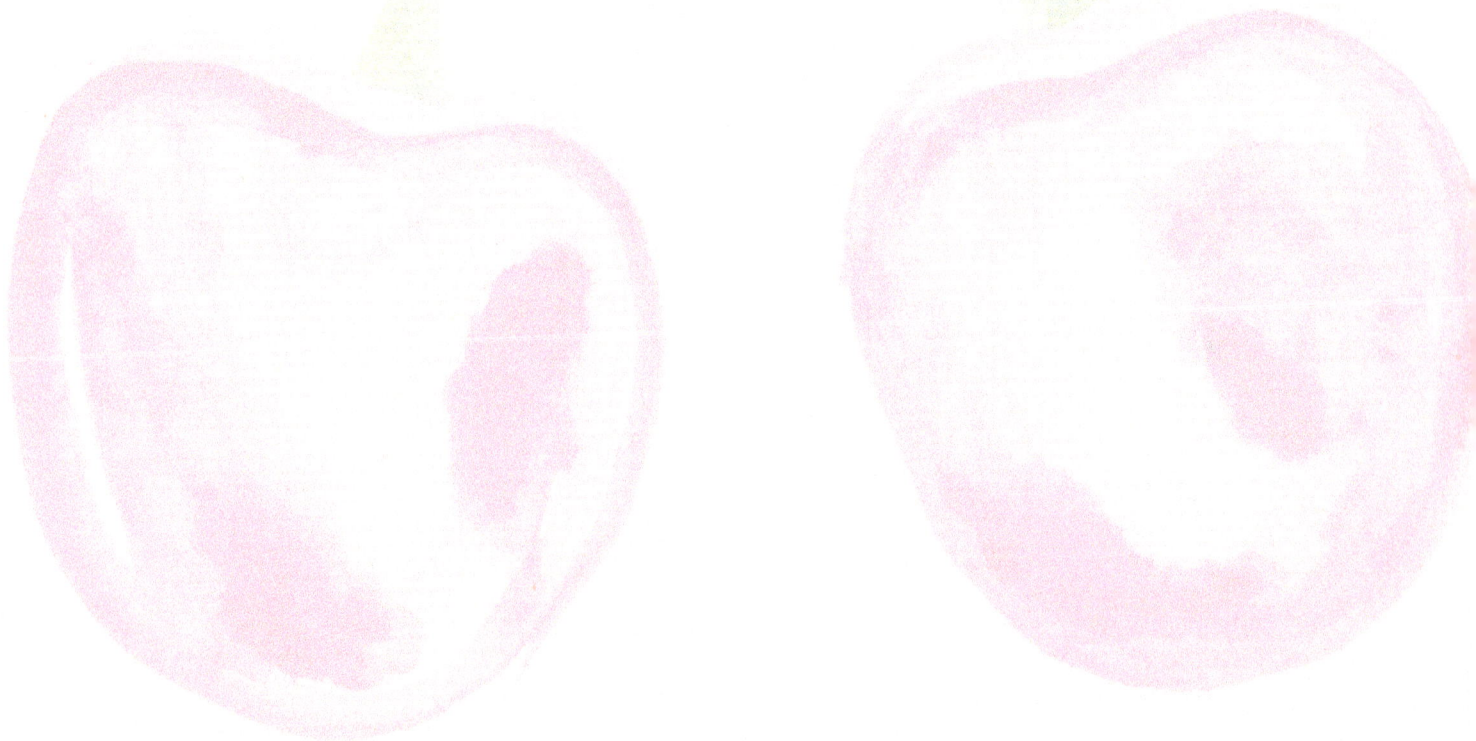

Internal Winter–The Organ's Alchemy

Day 1– Kidney: The first day of your bleed cleanses your kidneys. They are paired with your bladder. It awakens the element of water in your body. As the waters of winter descend on your cycle, the blood starts flowing and the kidneys awaken. Themes arise as your Kidney cleanses; Kidneys are your securities in life. They are inherited from your parents. You get your left kidney from your mother and your right from your father. Kidneys are your reproductive and your vitality organs. When you rest, these batteries can rest. If you live your life fast and hard, your kidneys will deplete just as fast. Tantra, an esoteric yogic tradition, believes the kidneys hold your Ojas. Ojas is your vitality, sexuality, and life force. In Taoism, your kidneys hold your dharma. This is your soul work, your life path that you are meant to align with. When your kidneys are imbalanced, you'll feel a lack of life force, have inner and outer fears, perhaps of not being able to provide for yourself or meet your needs. These feelings can show up on the first day of your bleed as irregularities in the blood, big emotional movements, and physical symptoms as well. Then let's talk fractals – if it's winter and you're cycling on your first day, you are a double dose of dark winter. You'll experience potent kidney energy as things may become louder. This is an opportunity to go deep within, become soulful, and nourish your deepest securities. Pay attention to which season of the year you are in, as that same season's organ will be even more activated. In harmony, kidneys are offer clarity. It is you engaging your willpower to go out into the planet with purpose and a soul-filled mission. The five elements are patterned in all things.

Day 2– Liver: The liver is expressed on day two of your bleed. It receives its nutrients from the health of the kidneys from the first day because in the five-element cycle, the kidneys mother the liver. The liver is the first yang season; It has an infantile energy to it in which is the energy of sunrise, the first growth sprouting, and new life emerging. Its energy shoots up, and without a balanced liver, it can burst out in anger and rage. Your liver looks out through the eyes during the day and draws the line of your sight.

The liver works with angles of perception; it shows you that it's all in the mind. Head one direction, you'll see certain things; Head in another direction, you'll see other things. Your mind is creating all of it. Which way will you walk? Your blood rests in your liver at night and is responsible for your dreams. Your dreams converse with your spirit. They whisper to you what you are here to do, and give you the vision to see the path you are walking. When your liver is imbalanced, you will feel very impulsive. Like the energy of spring, you will feel rage, anger, and impatience. This can be internal or external. Too much liver heat, and you will become explosive. Make a tea of milk thistle, oat straw, dandelion, and plantain to support this organ. In harmony, the liver imparts patience. It is you, envisioning your soul-led path and listening to the whispering of your dreams so you can start every day with the patience to know that it is all coming. These are the themes that arise during day two of your bleed.

Day 3- Heart: Your heart is cleansed on the third day. To connect with this organ on day three, use a seated movement to connect your pelvic floor to your heart to the crown of your head. This channels energy through your heart. The inhale is the uprising, the exhale the descending. The hands together strengthen the heart and connect you with YOU as the driver of your life. The palm is a miniature version of the heart; two palms together bring you into your third hand: the magician. The third day of your bleed is the summer of your bleed. It is the midpoint in your cycle where you pierce the center and begin making your way out. The heart is the center of your life; it works with your thymus gland and orients your vessel. Your heart works in your community through your hands. It is how you lend a hand and ask for a hand. It is also found in your tongue. Speech is an articulation of the heart, and if you ever have issues in your speech or stumble over your words, your heart is the root of this issue. When imbalanced, you could feel mania, overexcitement, and overzealousness. In Taoism, you are looking for everything in moderation. Even moderation. Your heart works with your small intestine to sort the pure from the impure and tells your spirit what to perceive joy from. Be careful what you take in; Your body doesn't discriminate- you need to. Your heart is fed when you give it the right people, experiences, and position yourself well in your community. The heart is participatory! In harmony, the heart imparts compassion. It is you receiving the messages from the heavens so you can perceive which path to follow in life, your soul's path. The path of your highest timeline.

Day 4- Spleen: The fourth day of your bleed is the late summer of your bleed. More seasons inside of seasons, inside of seasons! It cleanses the spleen. This organ gives you the focus you need to engage your will by experiencing the world through your senses. The spleen is the mind. It's your ability to exercise good judgment and hone your vision into appropriate action. It pivots the ethereal pieces of you into the tangible, actionable parts. It also shows up in your muscle quality. Muscles that are too lax create a mind that can't focus. Muscles too dense are an overly rigid mind. You want the flexibility to change course and remain strong. When imbalanced, worry arises. You'll have the tendency to overthink and overchew and not have anything to show for it. It's like analysis paralysis. If you're not in focused action, your spleen needs support. Support your spleen with good, wholesome foods and quality water. It's your postnatal qi (life force energy) and works with the stomach. Avoid processed sugar; It dampens the spleen and creates fog in the mind. Sitting and meditating is also medicine for the spleen; Consciously direct your thoughts. In harmony, the spleen gives you the gift of empathy. It focuses you on your path, and you can see life from other people's perspectives.

Day 5- Lungs: The fifth day of your bleed finishes off your menstrual cleanse. Although a longer bleed lengthens the time the organs are being impacted, Day five clears the lungs. This is the organ that directly works with the senses. It is the one organ impacted by the emotional experiences of the world. The lungs are where you hold your grief and sadness. They work in the season of autumn, and that is why they impart feelings of nostalgia. You get to reflect on the seasons of the light and bring your bounty into your home. When you repress emotions without allowing yourself to feel the full spectrum of your experience, the lungs are impacted. You hold on to life rather than let go of what you don't need. The lungs also work with the large intestine. When the lungs and large intestine are out of balance, you'll feel anxiety and will have trouble creating your life by design. You'll find yourself in your sympathetic nervous system response, a stress response known as "fight or flight." Support your lungs with breath-work, supporting the backs of the lungs with props in yoga, and take meditative walks in nature to take in the potency of the air. Let yourself laugh and cry and feel the full spectrum of the human experience. In harmony, the lungs will give you great courage in life to face your fears head-on, because now you know that to feel is to be seen in your experience. Only you can see yourself. You'll be more open to every experience so you can be made more whole; There is nothing to run away from!

Internal Spring
The Follicular Phase~ Growth and Renewal

Hormones: During this season, follicle-stimulating hormone (FSH) triggers the development of a mature egg, and estrogen levels gradually rise. This naturally higher-energy time is when you may feel more open to new experiences. Your hormones are still low, so the hemispheres of your brain can communicate more clearly. This is a nice time to intuitively map and plan out this new cycle you're beginning.

Cervical Release: As your egg starts to ripen, fluid becomes present. It normally appears cloudy, yellow, or white and feels sticky. You may also notice this fluid around the opening of your vagina. Yoni steams are a good practice to incorporate in this season to clear away any remains of the uterine lining and blood.

Energetics: Use this rise in energy to begin new tasks, pick back up on your to-do list, brainstorm ideas, learn, problem solve, start new projects, connect with friends, journal your daydreams, set intentions, and plan for this new cycle you're embarking on. Ease into this season and don't jump ahead of yourself to avoid burnout!

Move: This season is an ideal time for strength training and high-intensity workouts such as HIIT due to the increased energy. It may also feel good to dance, hike, swim, or bike. This time is about awakening after that winter cocoon.

Eat: The nutritional focus here is hormonal balance and egg maturation. Think Spring, eat green! Incorporate fermented foods, probiotics, and bitters to wake up digestion; Healthy fats are crucial for hormone production and help boost energy; Lean protein supports hormone balance and egg maturation by providing essential amino acids; Complete proteins and complex carbohydrates to support energy and hormone balance; Fresh veggies provide important vitamins and minerals to stabilize hormonal balance and overall nutrition.

Herbs: Bitter herbs, Nettle, Alfalfa, Dandelion Root, Red Clover, Damiana, Hawthorn, Matcha, Ginkgo, Gotu Kola, Oatstraw, Hibiscus, Spearmint, Rose Hips

Common Experiences: Energy rises, mood lifts and stability, higher focus, light or no cramps, breast tenderness decreases

Archetype: The *Mother* archetype is associated with this season. The *Mother* embodies the ideas of Maidenhood and manifests them in the real world. As your hormones and energy begin to rise again, you can be more practical and take action. The Mother energy invites us to be clearer-minded, optimistic, and ready to take on new things.

Internal Summer

The Ovulatory Phase~ Peak Energy and Fertility

Hormones: The ovaries take turns each month dropping the egg. This phase occurs when your mature egg is released, estrogen peaks, and is accompanied by a spike in testosterone levels. With the spike in estrogen, skin may appear thicker, juicier, and youthful. Fun fact: When one ovary is removed, the body's intelligence shifts to using the remaining one.

Cervical Release: Just before Ovulation, you should have the most fluids being released. It should appear clear and feel slippery like an egg white when stretched between your fingers. This fluid should last about four days, leading up to and at the time of ovulation. Yoni steams in this season can be helpful when you experience ovulation cramps (Mittelschmerz).

Energetics: In this season of life, you are magnetic. All things feel possible. Energy and manifesting feel at their peak. Script your desires and write. Be clear on what you do and don't want. Keep growing and be bold! The verbal and social centers of your brain are lit up in this season of your cycle. Your body craves community! This is a great time to schedule events, social gatherings, and important meetings. Confidence may be felt at this peak, and your brain is set for great communication skills. Have those important conversations and communicate boldly.

Move: Because your testosterone, estrogen, FSH (Follicle Stimulating Hormone), and LH (Luteinizing Hormone) are at peak, it may feel great to push your physical body and test your strength. Try HIIT, cycling, strength training, and cardio yoga. Get sweaty and feel that inner fire being stoked.

Eat: The nutritional focus in this phase should be to support ovulation and overall reproductive health. Eat healthy fats such as nuts to support hormone production; Lean protein supports energy levels during this high-energy phase; Antioxidant-rich berries support ovulation and overall reproductive health; Mixed greens provide essential vitamins and minerals; Seeds, nuts, and fruits symbolize fertility; Enjoy smoothies.

Herbs: Burdock Root, Nettle, Vitex/Chaste Berry, Red Clover, Dong Quai, Red Raspberry Leaf, Evening Primrose Oil, Milk Thistle Seed, Maca, Ashwagandha, Ginger, Shatavari, Rose Petals, Damiana, Cacao, Lemon Balm

Common Experiences: Mittelschmerz is the term that describes Ovulation pain, and is the pain of the egg popping out of the ovary and sliding into the fallopian tube. This is the peak point of ovulation. This pain isn't a concern as it is telling you exactly what your egg is doing. You may also notice breast fullness, increased basal body temperature, heightened senses, elevated mood, increased libido, enhanced creativity, and focus.

Archetype: The *Maga* archetype is associated with this season. The *Maga* embodies heightened confidence, a magnetic presence, and clear communication skills. This energy reminds us of our power and that expressing our desires isn't selfish but necessary for living in our full potential and inspiring others to do the same.

Internal Autumn

The Luteal Phase~ Preparation and Reflection

Hormones: Progesterone rises during this time, preparing your body for the possibility of pregnancy. If the fertilized egg doesn't become implanted, progesterone levels will fall, leading to the next menstrual phase. In your Inner Autumn, your body waits to see if the egg is fertilized. Progesterone increases, estrogen fluctuates, and testosterone decreases. Metabolism speeds up after the drop, which is where the excessive hunger comes from. You might feel emotional or have pre-period symptoms, which come from the hormonal fluctuations. Hormone balance through diet is key in this season to prevent PMS symptoms.

Cervical Release: After the peak of ovulation, you may notice there is far less fluid. It will become sticky and cloudy again and eventually go away, leading to more dry days preceding Moontime (bleed). It is a nice time to do a Yoni Steam to support potential cramps and create space for self-nourishment.

Energetics: Prioritize self-care, mental health, and practice healthy boundaries. Think guest of the party rather than the host. This phase is best for tasks requiring concentration and preparation, like finalizing projects or organizing. You are wrapping up your cycle. Pay attention to the irritants as they are keys to where you can improve your self-care and boundaries. Prioritizing balance between your to-dos and relaxation can support PMS and that inner fire I like to call the "Mood-eal" phase. Get prepared to slow down so that when Inner Winter hits, you can glide into the moon cocoon with more ease rather than experience a big crash. This preparation also helps create space for the incoming wisdom that will emerge during menstruation. Wind down.

Move: If you're feeling extra spicy in this season, a run or workout may be helpful to move that energy. Meditate and focus on breathing with techniques such as Breath of Fire. Your nervous system capacity is shifting here. Be kind to yourself and know you're just riding a wave and the world's really not ending. It is just a phase.

Eat: The nutritional focus in this season is hormonal balance and managing PMS symptoms and mood. Support food cravings by choosing snacks rich in healthy fats and high protein; Red meat is a great source of iron which can help prepare for menstrual bleeding; Lentils provide iron and fiber; Foods with anti-inflammatory properties to help manage cramping; Foods rich in B vitamins and healthy fats can support mood and hormonal balance; Foods rich in omega-3 fatty acids, which promote heart health, have anti-inflammatory properties and support brain function and overall well-being; Complex carbohydrates provide sustained energy; Antioxidants, particularly vitamin C, help protect cells and support a healthy immune system. Avoid or slowly wind down the caffeine intake, as this can lead to heightened anxiety during this sensitive time.

Herbs: Skullcap, Valerian, Tulsi, Chamomile, Yarrow, Red Raspberry Leaf, Nettle, Red Clover, Lavender, Lemon Balm, Chaste Tree (Vitex) Berry, Black Cohosh, Blue Vervain, Ginger, Cinnamon, Spearmint, Rose Petals, Cacao, Milky Oats, Oatstraw

Common Experiences: Breast tenderness, cramping, irritability, emotional sensitivity, bloating and water retention, mild weight gain, fatigue, slower digestion, mood swings, cravings for sweets or carbohydrates, mild aches and tension, lowered motivation, and difficulty focusing are all common in this season of life. Remember to be gentle with yourself and set boundaries so you can nurture what your body is asking for. Use these symptoms as an invitation to slow tend and give yourself what you need. These experiences are common, but it is not normal to feel so extreme. The experiences here help us notice what needs tending to, whether it's our hormone levels, diet, or lifestyle. This season of life is potent and holds many opportunities to stand in your Truth.

Archetype: The *Crone* archetype is associated with this season. The *Crone* embodies a time of evaluation, strategic planning, and boundary setting. The "PMS irritability" may often be dismissed and shamed, but it is really a time of discernment of what is and isn't working. Your inner wisdom is guiding you to declutter emotionally and physically for the highest good. The *Crone* sees through the illusions, and we are invited to speak our truths with compassion.

Journaling Through Your Cycle

A practice I have developed is that on the first day of my bleed, the start of a new cycle, I create a new Note in my phone with the date my bleed came. Like some people choose a word they want to embrace for the year, I have one for each cycle. Since this has been in practice, it has developed to where I can just hear the word and feel security in knowing that the word will be my theme for the incoming cycle.

I will also note when my bleed ended so I know when I started my Inner Spring, when I feel I'm in my Inner Summer, and when I feel the shift into my Inner Autumn. This helps me keep track of seasonal lengths and overall cycle length so I can book out my "month" and tells me if/how I can show up for my obligations. I can now tell when my Inner Winter will be and intentionally schedule myself unavailable for things. It has given me freedom in knowing I can really lock in for three solid weeks, and then I will have time carved out for myself.

This note serves as my cycle journal. By practicing this, I now see patterns in when I create my to-dos for the cycle, my emotional and reflective entries, how and when I feel some type of way about my relationships (reflecting on if I'm in my inner Autumn and if it's really the hormones talking), all my creative ideas, and when my intuition is speaking loud and clear. I then copy and paste all these into a document to review later.

At this point, since I have been doing this for a few years, my document is over 100 pages long. I like to read through it and see what ideas I have completed, or could be inspired by if I haven't completed, and emotions I have cycled through or kept repeating. As a business owner, it is also really fun to see all the social media posts I have come up with by noting them in each monthly cycle journal page.

You will be amazed at how long a cycle truly is and all the different emotions we move through each month. Having something to look back at amazes me at the evolution I receive each month. Being a cycling woman is truly incredible! I look forward to what will open for you in the process.

Daily Check-In

Journaling thoughts and feelings experienced throughout each month is an act of self-love and provides clarity, while fostering resilience against mood-related challenges faced during specific times throughout one's own unique journey! Below, important things to track each day are starred. The remaining prompts are optional and can be used to spark inspiration. Try to pick a few that feel relevant/important for the day and follow for 13 Moons (1 Lunar Year).

*Date: *External Moon Phase:

*Day of Cycle, Internal Phase: *Basal Body Temp:

*Cervical Fluid:

*What was my energy level today?

*What did I eat today?

*What does my inner weather feel like today?

What behaviors did I notice within myself today?

*What are a few words to distill my day?

What am I needing more or less of?

What was my sense of humor?

Where was my mind today?

What creative ideas came today?

How can the place I'm in today serve my project?

Symbols, illustrations, colors, shapes that describe my day:

What dreams did I have last night?

How do I feel about my partner? (if applicable)

42

Use this chart to record words you feel throughout a cycle to recognize recurring themes

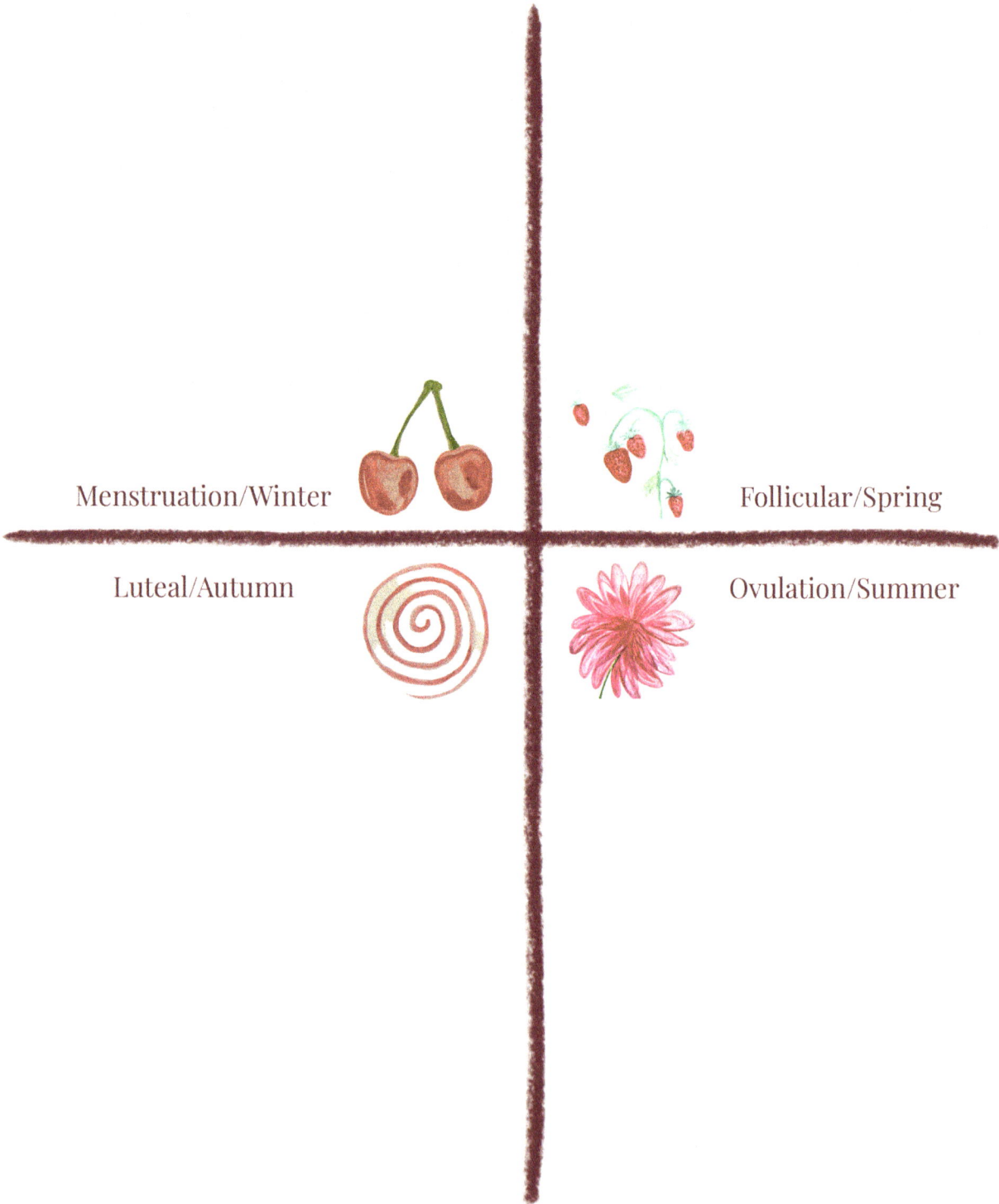

Menstruation/Winter

Follicular/Spring

Luteal/Autumn

Ovulation/Summer

① Basal Body Temperature Tracking Chart

Dates covered:

cycle Number:

DAY OF CYCLE:	1	2	3	4	5	6	7	8	9	10	11	12	13	14	15	16	17	18	19	20	21	22	23	24	25	26	27	28	29	30	31	32	33	34	35	36	37
DATE:																																					
TIME:																																					
99°F																																					
98.9°F																																					
98.8°F																																					
98.7°F																																					
98.6°F																																					
98.5°F																																					
98.4°F																																					
98.3°F																																					
98.2°F																																					
98.1°F																																					
98°F																																					
97.9°F																																					
97.8°F																																					
97.7°F																																					
97.6°F																																					
97.5°F																																					
97.4°F																																					
97.3°F																																					
97.2°F																																					
97.1°F																																					
97°F																																					
CERVICAL FLUID:																																					
SEX:																																					
FEVER:																																					
ALCOHOL:																																					

• CERVICAL RELEASE TYPES: B=Bleed, D=Dry, S=Sticky, E=Eggwhite (Fill each day with the corresponding letter.

• Leave an "X" on the days you're sexually active, because this affects the cervical fluid.

• Keep in mind, if you've drank alcohol or had a fever, this will affect your basal temperature. Write "A" or "F".

Cyclical Living Overview

Menstruation

• Carbs and starches • Bread • Pasta
• Easily digestible and warm foods
• Leafy Greens: Spinach, Kale, Lettuce, etc.
• Red Meat • Lentils • Beans • Eggs
• Healthy Fats/oils • Bone Broth • Fish • Nuts
• Miso • Carrots • Beets • Hearty Stews
• Mushrooms • Rice • Broccoli • Potatoes
• Pumpkin Seeds • Berries • Bell Peppers
• Dates • Dark Chocolate • Banana
• Grapes • Cherries • Squashes
• Cinnamon • Chia Seeds • Seeds
• Turmeric • Nutmeg • Ginger
• Fennel • Red Clover • Catnip
• Chamomile • Hawthorn
• Raspberry Leaf
• Cacao • Rose
• Passionflower
• Skullcap

Follicular

• Fermented Foods: Kimchi, Sauerkraut, Yogurt
• Eggs • Chicken • Beans • Lentils • Tofu
• Greens • Sprouts • Cabbage • Broccoli
• Brussel Sprouts • Quinoa • Carrots • Zucchini
• Artichoke • Cucumbers • Pickles • Peas • Oats
• Lemons • Limes • Oranges • Grapefruit
• Kiwi • Mangoes • Berries • Apples
• Brazil Nuts • Cashews • Chia Seeds
• Seeds • Flax Seeds • Healthy Fats
• Cilantro • Dill • Bitter Herbs
• Alfalfa • Ginkgo • Nettle
• Gotu Kola • Hawthorn
• Raspberry Leaf
• Dandelion
• Red Clover
• Matcha
• Damiana

Winter: Rest

• Light Stretching • Yin Yoga • Naps • Baths • Reading • Light Walks • Warrior Facemasks • Sauna • Flowy Art • Reflection Journaling

Your body is processing the shedding of your uterine lining. Rest is best here. The social vibe is almost non-existent at this time—at least for the first few days. Heavy exercise may cause stronger cramps so take it easy. Due to the decline in hormones, there is easier communication in the brain so intuition is clearer. Hydrate. Reflect. nourish!

Spring: Rebirth

• Core workouts • Walks • Strength Training • Vinyasa Yoga • Hikes • Bike • HIIT • Swim • Pilates • Creating To-Dos for this Cycle

As your energy starts to return, feel your body coming back into new life. The main hormones at play are slowly rising, so the hemispheres of your brain can still easily communicate. This time is for planning and brainstorming. Map out your goals for this cycle. Embrace this "spring"ing energy!

Autumn: Reflect

• Pelvic Floor Exercises • Hatha Yoga • Pilates • Hot Yoga • Sauna • Barre • HIIT • Reflective Journaling • Meditation • Breathwork

If the egg is not fertilized, Progesterone and Testosterone drop, and Estrogen fluctuates. Depending how they decrease, an imbalance can lead to PMS symptoms. Reduce external stress, notice the logic shifting and the triggers about boundaries and speaking Truth. Nurture self.

Summer: Radiate

• Cardio Yoga • Strength Training • HIIT • Cycling • Social Events • Get Sweaty • Hot Yoga • Swim • Running • Gratitude Journaling

This season your hormone levels are all peaking, allowing you to feel radiant. Script your desires, schedule important meetings & events. Embrace the magnetism that comes with feeling on top of the world. You are fertile and that can be applied to many areas of your life, not just to create a human but your dreams too.

Luteal

• Ginger
• Catnip
• Chamomile
• Raspberry Leaf
• Cinnamon • Nettle
• Lemon Balm • Rose
• Chasteberry/ Vitex
• Maple Syrup • Nut Butter
• Stewed Apples • Squashes
• Banana • Dates • Brussel Sprouts
• Sauteed veggies • Spinach
• Easily digestible foods • Carrots
• Avocados • Almonds • Healthy Fats
• Chia Seeds • Olive Oil • Beets • Parsnip
• Tahini • Pumpkin Seeds • Flax Seed • Turnips
• Dark Chocolate • Brown Rice • Walnuts • Barley
• Quinoa • Eggs • Sweet Potatoes • Legumes
• Chickpeas • Oats • Yogurt • Beans
• Turkey • Lentils • Chicken • Fish

Ovulation

• Ginger
• Turmeric
• Maca • Zinc
• Magnesium
• Shatavari • Iron
• Selenium • Dong Quai
• Green Tea • Red Clover
• Vitex/Chasteberry • Nettle
• Damiana • Raspberry Leaf
• Lemon Balm • Apples • Bananas
• Turnips • Beets • Chard • Kale
• Pumpkin Seeds • Carrots • Parsnips
• Celery • Cucumber • Broccoli • Avocado
• Dark Leafy Greens • Spinach • Sweet Potatoes
• Melons • Berries • Dark Chocolate • Dates
• Nutritional Yeast • Olive Oil • Bell Peppers
• Whole Grains • Quinoa • Oats • Brazil Nuts
• Beans • Lentils • Cottage Cheese • Yogurt
• Eggs • Chicken • Legumes • Red Meat • Fish

45

Afterword

This guide is an invitation to connect deeper with your Menstrual Cycle. It was created with love for all the Women who came before us and who will come after us. It offers basic understandings that we should've been taught in school or from our Elders, but unfortunately, this knowledge has been stripped from us. It's so evident how much power our cycles hold, and the world would appear and feel so different if we were all taught this knowledge. It's really just a deep Re-Memberance back into the Wisdom we've always carried and is our Birthright to follow. This guide is not rigid and set in stone either. This practice brings awareness to your flow.

I share this guide from a heartfelt, passionate place. In my journey of reconnecting with my cycle, there are so many teachings. I'm grateful for the accessibility we have during this time to the internet, and that information is resurfacing. I have also earned a lot of this wisdom by simply listening and letting my body be the guide for what I'm experiencing.

You may notice I tended to repeat myself in this book, but that's because I feel so passionate and have many ways of saying the same thing. I also believe repetition helps integrate it into the logical mind and then seeps into the subconscious programming. This is how cyclical living has been in practice for me over the years. The chart on Page 45 demonstrates this visually and is a recreation of the one I've had hanging on my fridge. I encourage you to do the same.

The wisdom shared in this book comes from my experience over the last five years of reclaiming this Birthright. I hold deep gratitude for the numerous teachers who have already done work in this area. Their knowledge and wisdom have helped lay the groundwork for this guide. After countless hours of research, I still have never quite found a guide that encompasses and lays it all out in a way that is simple to understand. I hope this guide can give you the foundations to build this deep connection to yourself and watch it transform all areas of your life as it has for my experience, in my body.

A strong intention for this book is to share this wisdom in a simple, yet engaging way that young girls can understand the immense power they hold. This is a guide I wish I had at a younger age and now want to give back to girls as they walk through this initiation. I dream of a world where the language of this book is used to talk about this sacred transition and phase of life.

My hope is that while this guide has been laid out to be simple, it does not take away from the immense power of cycling. I want to change the idea that this cycle is a "burden to deal with" every month to a celebration and is deeper wisdom that our bodies hold.

If you are unfamiliar with cyclical living, this information can feel like cracking into a whole new world, but that's because it is. I have been sitting with this book for many moons waiting for the right time. But with each new cycle of mine, more information comes through. I decided to trust that what I share is enough, because it'll never be complete. This is infinite wisdom that comes with this awareness. I trust it is the right time, and what I present is enough to sync you into your own flow; a place where your own downloads will come through.

Welcome back home.

Dedications & Gratitude

I dedicate this book to my inner pre-teen who didn't have this wisdom at Menarche and now gets to learn, reclaim, and share this with others. To my (future) daughter and her daughters. May we continue to reclaim this inherent power together through our bloodline.

I dedicate this book to all the wise women before me, all those after me, and all the ones who walk with me at this potent time in her-story. May we reclaim what was stolen from us; May we re-member a world where we can live in balance and flow; May we never have to live separate from our superpower again.

Thank you to all the beautiful mirrors I've met along the way. The dear sisters who have taken the time to sit with this book while it was still in the phases of gestation. Thank you to the sisters who have encouraged me to follow my cycle and who do it alongside me. Thank you to my teachers who have protected this wisdom with all their hearts.

Thank you to my Grams, Karen Killbourne-Thiel, for all the Women's work you did in your lifetime through your paintings, sculptures, poetry, Women's circles, teaching, and for Planned Parenthood. You always remain an inspiration to weave my art into my work. I dedicate this book to you as a continuation of love for women and all that we are. Some of the art in this book was sketched by my Grams and painted by me. What a gift to follow her hands and co-create another project together.

Acknowledgements

I want to acknowledge all the beautiful humans who took the time to review my pre-release and offer their wisdom and support throughout my life. From family, to friends, to soul-family, you have all played a role in my expansion and hold a unique place in my heart. Each one of you has such special gifts to offer to the world at this time and deserve to be recognized, too.

To my love, *Dominick Phaller*. For always encouraging me to speak my truth. For embracing that I am a Cycling Womban. For not shaming, but celebrating me and all my phases. For listening to me with presence and teaching all your girl and guy friends about their "periods." For being a Divine man of love and Truth and always having my back. It is such a blessing to be building this life together hand in hand!

To *Marjorie Klimek*, my dear momma, for bringing me Earthside and supporting me with so much love in every phase of my growth. It is an incredible blessing to have you as my Mother in this lifetime. Thank you for reading and re-reading this book countless times and always answering when I call and text with compassion, and making it so evident how proud of me you are. Your belief in me is such potent fuel to my fire.

To *Jayda Lee Jean*, my infinite Soul Sister. For being a witness to me in this lifetime and all those before and after this one. What a gift it is to be riding the same wavelength with you, no matter the time or distance. For writing such a beautiful foreword attesting to the power of being a woman and our sisterhood. For inspiring me to include a page on Skin Cycling and sharing your embodied wisdom that came from your own skin journey. For sharing your photography skills in collaboration to add another layer of story-telling to this book. For all your beautiful gifts you offer this world and beyond: www.eternity-rising.com.

To *Madison Vinje*, "a ceremonialist and devotee of the primordial feminine. She helps guide women into a remembrance of their inherent shamanic nature, medicine, Eros, and soul." You have done just that for me, my dear sister. Thank you for shining a light on my blind spots to help me uncover some of my deepest soul-desires. For nudging me to fearlessly talk about Birth Control and how it directly correlates to the disruption of our organic nature and our Liberation. For sharing your medicine with me and guiding me through the medicine wheel with the sacred Deer, Bear, Wolf, and Snake to unleash my voice and feral nature. AhOoo!

To *Jin Dalsin*, Spiritual Guide and Channel for Orin Speaks- www.OrinSpeaks.com. For guiding my spirit and flesh when I feel lost or stuck. For your endless encouragement and your vision in the unseen. Your guidance has helped shape me and redirect me on my purposeful path, time after time.

To *Samantha Scott*, PhD- Mother, Author, Spiritual Facilitator, and Moon Sister of mine. For always encouraging me to look at and take things deeper and see the sacredness in all of life and death. For being a "big sister," I never had and journeying through the Perfection Houses with me. For holding the space for so many others at your studio, Event Horizon, and sharing your art through Atma Healings.

To *Lily Alvarez*, Practitioner of KaHuna Medicine, Yoga, and Sound Healing, and my dear Moon Sister. For sharing your heart with me and learning to dance in this life together. Literally and figuratively. For practicing cyclical living with me and embodying our inherent nature, normalizing the language around it all. For holding the space for me in transitional times through your incredible Kahuna Medicine, yoga, and sound healing classes. For holding space with me for the women under the Full and New Moons for a Lunar Year. This book was conceived under the Leo Full Moon with the help of Trumpet Vine and Sunflower Essences. How special!

To *Eric Ament-Two Rivers* of Anahata Herbals, for taking one look at my book in its baby stages and nudging me to use my own art instead of the pre-made watercolor graphics. I giggled when he said this because before the conversation, I was not a fan of watercolor. Thanks to my sweet friend Hannah Frodge, who's an incredible watercolor artist, I came to find out it was all because I was using the wrong materials! This challenge opened a whole new medium for me to explore and to connect with my grandmother, Karen, who was a master at watercolor. Some of the illustrations are co-creations between her and me as I discovered her sketchbooks and painted in the lines of what she left behind.

To *Gigi Stafne*, of Green Wisdom of Natural and Botanical Medicine. For seeing me eye to eye and believing in me so deeply. For being a mirror of the Wise Woman within. For the endless words of encouragement in all my projects over the years. For all the work you do across the Midwest and beyond. For being the bridge for SO many humans to remember their connection to this Earth's cycles, the plants, and each other.

To *Al Wallace*, my Moon Sister. For your design eyes making sure all the elements flowed throughout the book. For the squishy hugs and smiles you bring me at the right times and places. For the sisterhood and warmth you bring to our Libra Moon sign connection.

To *Allicia Speich*, my Herbal Sister. For your endless knowledge and curiosity about what our changing bodies are experiencing. For your love and support as my colleague and friend. For all the work you're doing in the realm of Women's Health, especially tending to the Mother and Baby.

To *Amelia Chapman,* Female Nervous System Practitioner. (Instagram *@ameliaunfolding*). For being so intentional in all that you do. For always inviting me to be mindful and to pause in the present to breathe into my body. For all the work you're doing in the world of Women's Health and being a lighthouse for so many to come home to our bodies.

To *Mary Lou Singleton*, Herbalist, Nurse Practitioner, and Midwife of Enchanted Family Medicine. It was so special to listen to you speak so passionately in your class, *"Riding Your Cycle,"* at the Midwest Women's Herbal Conference 2025. I felt so deeply inspired and empowered by witnessing you share this wisdom.

To *Kat Villain*, whom I learned about the body's alchemy during menstruation. This felt like such an important piece of wisdom to share and created an even deeper meaning to the transformation we go through during menstruation!

To *Nicole LeBlanc Paulson*, my most influential high school English teacher. For your endless encouragement in my writings, no matter the topic. For showing up as authentically you. You taught all of us hormonal teenagers how to take a "Mindful Minute" at the start of each class and has always stuck with me. It was such an exciting full circle to share this book with you as one of my first readers because I never thought I'd be an author, and here we are with my first book!

To *Jill Bellefeuille*, a student of the Source of all that is and founder of Soul Voyager Holistic Healing. For helping me refine my language skills and navigate the English language with all your English teacher edits. For being such a bright light and reminding me to do the same in spaces that feel dimming.

To *Breana Crotteau,* founder of KIEPO Solutions and HWS Cannabis Company. For all your encouragement in sharing all my mediums of offerings and inspiring me to anchor into my small town. For all the work you're doing for the rural communities. For connecting me to *Julie Jo Larson,* an experienced author, who then led me to *Krista Soukup* of Blue Cottage Agency. Together, these two helped me get to the finish line with this book.

To *Cheryl Reitan,* an accomplished writer and author, for encouraging me from the start. For being a mentor in a whole new world for me (the author world).

Index

Broster, Alice. *"Period Blood Color Chart: What You Need To Know."* 2025, March 13, https://flo.health/menstrual-cycle/health/period/period-blood-color.

GoodMindAndBody. *"How To Plan Your Life Around Your Cycle."* 2024, November 12, https://goodmindandbody.com/how-to-plan-your-life-around-your-cycle/.

Guan, BreAnna. *"11 Foods That Boost Ovulation and Improve Hormone Health Naturally."* https://drbreannaguan.com/foods-that-boost-ovulation/.

Harju, Deborah. *"How to Choose the Right Clay for Your Skin Type."* 2023, May 18, https://helloglow.co/right-clay-for-your-skin-type/.

Jay, Shani. *"Sacred Bleeding: White Moon & Red Moon Cycles Explained."* https://revoloon.com/shanijay/052020-white-moon-and-red-moon-cycles.

Johansson, Steve. *"Cycle Syncing Food Chart: Eat Your Way to Happy Hormone."* https://www.mothersalwaysright.com/cycle-syncing-food-chart-guide/.

Juta. *"The History of The Calendar."* 2020, https://www.livingwiththemoon.com/the-history-of-the-calendar/.

Lee, Angela Ryan. *"How Basal Body Temperature Relates to Fertility."* 2024, September 14, https://www.verywellhealth.com/basal-body-temperature-5210908.

Lee, Jema. *"Menstrual Cycle Archetypes 101: Maiden, Mother, Maga & Crone."* 2025, July 2. https://cyclicalschool.com/menstrual-cycle-archetypes-101-maiden-mother-maga-crone/

Pires de Lima, Teresa. *"Menstrual Cycle Food Chart."* 2023, October 23, https://elara.care/nutrition/menstrual-cycle-food-chart/.

Planned Parenthood. *"What's The Cervical Mucus Method of FAMs."* https://www.plannedparenthood.org/learn/birth-control/fertility-awareness/whats-cervical-mucus-method-fams.

Sundays, Seaside. *"16 Fertility Herbs To Help You Get Pregnant Fast."* 2018, July 2, https://seasidesundays.com/fertility-herbs/.

The Business of Birth Control. Executive Producers: Abby Epstein and Ricki Lake, Documentary, Gaia TV, 2021.

The Moon School. *"A Guide to Menstrual Rituals: 13 Best Ways to Honor Your Sacred Blood Cycle."* https://www.themoonschool.org/menstruation/menstrual-rituals/.

Young, Kayla. *"11 Amazing Herbals For Facial Steaming."* 2023, July 23, https://luxeluminous.com/herbs-for-facial-steaming/.

About The Author

Zoë Klimek is an author, herbalist, artist, birthworker, and holistic guide based in the forests of Northern Minnesota. Her journey has taken her across the West Coast and into the heart of Hawaii, where she experienced a profound reconnection with the land, the rhythms of nature, and the sacred path of birthwork. It was there that her soul truly came alive.

During her time on the Big Island, surrounded by lush landscapes and the warmth of her host family, Zoë felt deeply connected to the Earth's vitality and flow. Yet, beneath the beaming sun, she began to long for something unexpected~ the stillness of home. Missing her first Minnesota winter left her soul homesick for the quiet, reflective power of the cold. When she returned in January, the heart of winter, she made a vow to stop resisting the season and instead honor its wisdom, and to romanticize the cycles of life, even in their dormancy. With that vow has come many powerful lessons, one of them being that women experience four seasons within a moon cycle on top of the four seasons lead by the sun.

Her personal healing journey, experience of quitting hormonal birth control, and learning to embrace the wisdom of her menstrual cycle transformed her life. Now, she shares that transformation with others, offering knowledge, support, and soulful tools to help people reconnect with their own cyclical nature and birthright.

She supports women through herbal consultations, cycle syncing guidance, yoni steaming formulations, and holistic women's health practices (which can be found at www.thecyclicalwomban.com), Rooted in her deep connection to the Earth, Zoë also creates art and jewelry from natural materials such as bones and crystals, honoring the cycles of life, death, and renewal through her creative work.

Zoë writes with the same intention she lives: to honor the wisdom of the body, the beauty of the Earth, and the seasons that shape us all.

www.ingramcontent.com/pod-product-compliance
Lightning Source LLC
Chambersburg PA
CBHW061223270326
41927CB00024B/3481